A GUIDE TO CONFLICT FREE CONNECTION

A comprehensive guide to creating harmony at home, avoiding issues with your spouse, and being in a relationship without the nagging and fighting.

Daniel Tucker

Table of contents

INTRODUCTION

The power of peaceful partnership.

For what reason do a few homes feel loaded with harmony and others don't? How might you make a harmony filled home and for what reason is it so significant?

As far as I can tell I find that when an individual or family is focused in understanding and in Christ, Harmony is available. Sure a home could feel tranquil due to the magnificence or quietness or a delightful view, however I accept those qualities alone don't achieve harmony.

What is harmony: Harmony is independence from brutality from peers, accomplices, family, outsiders, and the state. Harmony is sympathy for other people. Harmony is having the option to develop and flourish and be what your identity is. Harmony is independence from double ideas and thinking.

What is the significance of harmony in the family?

- For building love in the family.

- knowing the qualities that a family values.

- Helps increment concordance and harmony among all relatives.

- Assists, keep dreading away from the youngsters.

- Advances sound living.

A fundamental piece of everyday life is to think about what is esteemed in the family. Kids are not befuddled when they comprehend and realize what is generally significant, and feel regarded. Having quiet organization in the family, assists the kids with filling together as one and makes life more and better.

Chapter 1

Understanding Triggers

What constitutes a trigger? A trigger is a prompt that induces a response, commonly associated with something that initiates or exacerbates certain symptoms.

Exploring Triggers within the Family

In the context of family dynamics, when a family member becomes a trigger, the optimal course of action is to prioritize self-honoring and refocus on personal needs. Consider what you require at that moment for your well-being. It might involve expressing to the individual that their comments are unwelcome and requesting them to cease. Alternatively, it could entail stepping away from the situation, or engaging in a sincere one-on-one conversation on a different occasion, delving into the root of their comments. Whatever path you choose, commence and conclude with self-compassion.

How can one navigate family situations that lead to unnecessary triggers?

- Identify your personal stress signals.
- Allocate time for activities that bring personal meaning, relaxation, and enjoyment for both you and your family.
- Incorporate deep breathing or mindfulness techniques.
- Prioritize adequate sleep.
- Acknowledge and accept your emotions and feelings.
- Take into account the emotional needs of your family members.

Why do triggers manifest so readily?

Easily feeling triggered can stem from diverse factors such as past experiences, trauma, stress, anxiety, or other mental health conditions.

It's crucial to identify your emotional triggers and enlist the assistance of a mental health professional. They can aid in crafting coping mechanisms and delving into the root causes.

What's the strategy for managing emotional triggers?

Be aware of your immediate reactions, linking emotions with physical sensations. Take breaks, delve into the emotions, work with a professional, prioritize self-care, engage in mindfulness and meditation, establish a grounding routine, and set healthy boundaries.

How can I maintain control during triggering moments?

In moments of heightened emotion, deploy relaxation techniques. Practice deep-breathing exercises and employ imaginative exercises to regain composure.

Create a soothing environment, or recite a calming word like "Relax." Incorporate activities like listening to music, journaling, or practicing a few yoga poses, whatever fosters a sense of relaxation. Actively engage in these practices and strive to steer clear of anger-inducing situations.

Chapter 2

The art of active listening

The idea may appear straightforward, yet engaging in active listening—wholeheartedly concentrating on the speaker's words—requires dedication and refinement through practice.

Being an active listener involves earnestly striving to comprehend the speaker's emotions, thoughts, and intentions. It entails directing one's thoughts entirely toward the speaker, prioritizing understanding over formulating one's response.

What are the five principles of active listening?

- Dedicate your complete attention to the speaker and acknowledge their message.
- Demonstrate that you are genuinely listening.
- Offer constructive feedback.
- Withhold judgment.

- Respond appropriately to the speaker's communication.

Why is active listening a vital skill in family communication?

Active listening serves as an effective means to enhance communication within a family. It communicates genuine interest in what your child has to share, fostering a deeper connection. To practice active listening, devote your complete attention to your child.

How can I employ active listening within my family?

- Maintain direct eye contact and face the speaker, reinforcing a sense of familial connection.

- Refrain from interruptions: In family discussions, avoid interrupting in a manner you wouldn't appreciate. Stay composed and understanding until it's your turn to speak.

- Listen without passing judgment or hastily drawing conclusions.

- Avoid preemptively planning your response: Concentrate on the speaker without letting your mind wander elsewhere.

- Refrain from imposing your opinions or solutions: Acknowledge your family's feelings and avoid imposing your views on them.

- Maintain focus: Dedicate your attention solely to them in that moment.

- Pose questions: Once the person has finished speaking, engage in a dialogue by asking questions and collaboratively reaching conclusions.

As a child, permit your parents to convey their thoughts before offering your response.

Avoid interrupting them in the midst of a sentence, especially if you disagree; instead, wait until they have fully expressed their thoughts.

What advantages come from listening to your parents?

Listening to your parents holds numerous benefits. Given their intimate knowledge of you, parents possess unparalleled insight into your needs. Throughout your growth, they have provided care—feeding you, clothing you, and tending to your needs. As a child, embracing the act of listening to them proves to be one of the most valuable aspects of your upbringing.

Chapter 3

Mindful Communication Techniques

What is Mindful Communication?

Mindful communication encompasses the application of mindfulness principles to our interactions with others. These principles encompass setting an intention, maintaining complete presence, fostering openness and non-judgment, and engaging with others through compassion and wisdom.

Our connections with others are not always mindful.

The appropriate approach to communication involves embracing mindfulness. Mindful communication entails being fully present, actively engaged, and open-minded. This approach enhances relationships and diminishes stress by fostering deeper understanding, empathy, and respect.

Practicing mindful communication urges you to actively listen to others, promoting a more profound and enriching exchange of ideas and understanding.

Exploring this non-judgmental approach opens the door to profound learning and insight. It enables you to consider new perspectives, adopt objectivity amidst conflicts, and evolve into the empathetic person you aspire to be.

What are the three facets of mindful communication?

- **Presence**: Anchoring our awareness in the body.
- **Intention**: Cultivating a heartfelt orientation to comprehend our emotions.
- **Attention**: Training to concentrate on specific aspects of our experience for a more profound perspective.

Failure to engage in mindful verbal expression gives rise to misunderstandings, conflicts, and stress, underscoring the importance of adopting a mindful communication approach.

Highlighting our relationships in a negative light, ineffective communication can lead to detrimental consequences. Conversely, proficient communication fosters positive outcomes such as heightened awareness, mindfulness, and attentiveness.

Inadequate communication skills not only contribute to anxiety, depression, and stress in adults but also make them susceptible to social isolation and loneliness, potentially causing harm or disrupting family unity.

Chapter 4

Navigating disagreement with empathy

In the process of resolving conflicts, empathy plays a crucial role by enabling individuals to view the situation from the other person's perspective and comprehend their point of view. This fosters the establishment of rapport and contributes to a more positive and constructive atmosphere for resolution.

Empathizing with one another serves to diminish negative emotions like anger, frustration, or resentment that often act as catalysts for conflicts, escalating them into arguments or fights. Additionally, empathy facilitates the identification of common ground, underlying issues, and the generation of solutions that mutually satisfy both parties.

Experiencing empathy doesn't require conformity, but it necessitates a willingness to understand and reach agreements in order to foster harmonious resolutions.

It's straightforward,

- **Sympathy** involves comprehending your own perspective or experience in relation to someone else's.
-
- **Empathy** involves understanding someone else's perspective or experience.

How can you approach conflict with empathy?

- Offering apologies holds significant weight.
- Engage in active listening.
- Empathize by putting yourself in their shoes.
- Express gratitude and appreciation.
- In essence, practicing empathy is a key to resolving most conflicts.

Handling Individuals Lacking Empathy

- Avoid taking their anger or judgments personally.
- Refrain from attempting to make them understand your feelings.

- Foster connections with individuals you trust.
- Understand that your worth is not contingent on their approval.

Chapter 5

Establishing Healthy Boundaries

Establishing healthy boundaries supports the development of self-control in young people, fostering their sense of belonging within the family and society, and creating a feeling of being cared for and secure. These boundaries are essential not only for the well-being of the young individuals but also for parents to effectively care for themselves and other family members. Boundaries serve as guidelines delineating appropriate behavior and responsibilities in relationships.

The key lies in being assertive, meaning being firm yet not aggressive in asserting your own rights, needs, and boundaries while considering those of others. Assertiveness entails effectively communicating your points with both firmness and fairness, incorporating empathy. An integral aspect of assertiveness involves the practice of politely but firmly saying **"No."**

Setting a boundary is essentially about expressing your needs and expectations clearly and effectively.

During this process, it can be crucial to tactfully address someone's hurtful behavior, although it shouldn't be the primary focus. Emphasizing what someone has done wrong may trigger defensiveness. Instead, initiate the conversation by expressing how you feel and stating your needs.

How can I establish and uphold effective boundaries?
- Begin with a few well-defined boundaries.
- Reflect on the rationale behind your boundaries.
- Contemplate establishing boundaries early on.
- Strive for consistency in maintaining your boundaries.
- Allocate dedicated time for yourself.
- Implement healthy boundaries, especially on social media.

How can I establish boundaries within my family?

- Take time for introspection.
- Communicate your boundaries calmly and clearly.
- When someone breaches a boundary, allow them an opportunity to make amends.
- Place a priority on your own self-care.
- Respect the boundaries set by other family members.
- Recognize that this is an ongoing process.

As a young individual, how can I establish healthy boundaries with my parents?

- Familiarize yourself with your rights as a child.
- Reflect on what holds significance for you.
- Practice assertiveness.
- Demonstrate respect.
- Exercise patience.
- Build a support network.
- Consider seeking professional assistance.

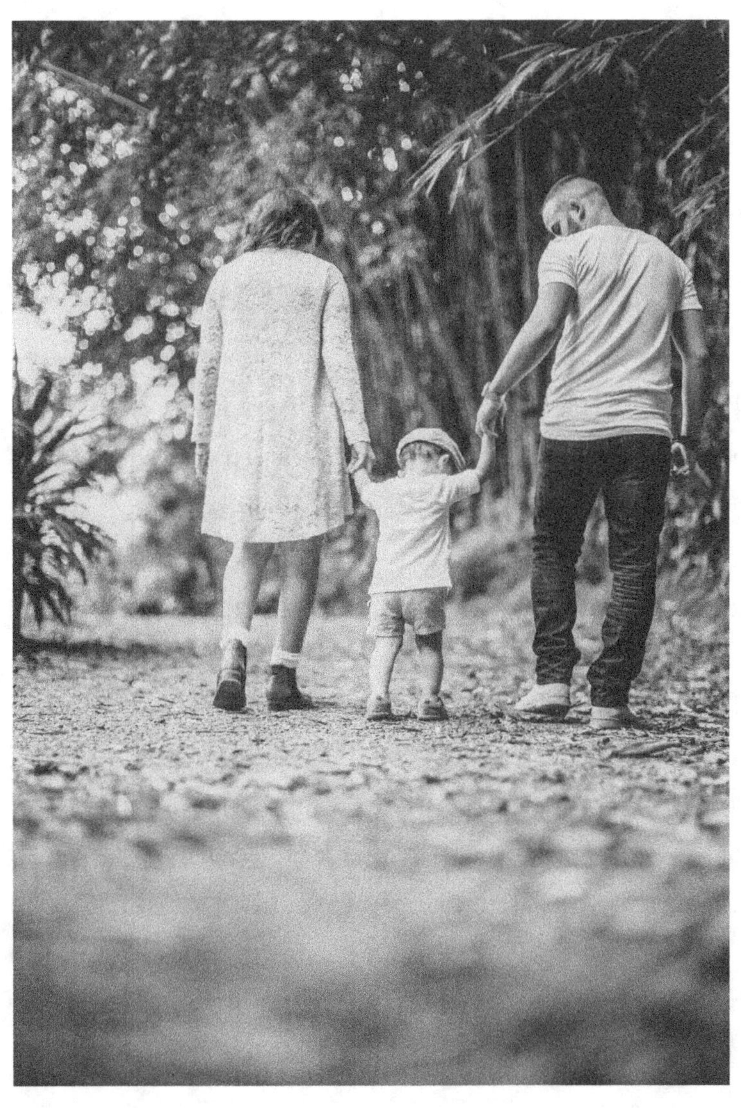

Chapter 6

Collaborative Problem solving

Engaging in collaborative problem-solving entails the cognitive processing of an individual, involving both cognitive and social skills.

This approach eschews the utilization of power, control, and motivational techniques. Instead, it emphasizes collaboration with family members and friends to address issues that may lead to unmet expectations and concerning behavior.

The practice of collaborative problem-solving has the potential to enhance the parent-child relationship. Through joint efforts to find solutions, parents and children foster a sense of teamwork and trust. This collaborative approach contributes to building a stronger bond between parents and children, fostering a greater sense of connection for the children with their parents.

How to address Unresolved Issues?

Commence by gathering information and comprehending your child's perspective on the matter. This initial step involves active listening, validating emotions, and expressing genuine curiosity. Clearly convey your concerns and needs related to the situation.

Collaborative Problem Solving (CPS) serves as a communication method that aids a child or young person in developing problem-solving skills while supporting cognitive and social-emotional development. The emphasis lies in collaborative dialogue rather than imposing solutions.

How can I navigate family issues?
- Strive to maintain composure.
- Attempt to set emotions aside.
- Refrain from interrupting when someone is speaking.
- Engage in active listening to understand both their words and intentions.

- Ensure your comprehension by posing questions to confirm understanding.
- Express your perspective transparently and truthfully.

Chapter 7

Cultivating Appreciation

Initiate and conclude with purpose. Each morning, reflect on what you value and anticipate for the day, and as you retire for the night, acknowledge everything you're thankful for. Maintain continuous awareness throughout the day, identifying small things for which you can express gratitude.

Fostering gratitude involves the intentional choice to direct your time and attention toward appreciation, a pivotal factor in influencing your overall experience and, ultimately, your well-being.

Encourage every family member, spanning from the youngest to the eldest, to share one thing they appreciate each day. Whether it's a sibling's kind gesture or the beauty of nature, this routine assists in acknowledging and valuing the positive aspects of our lives.

How do I show appreciation to my family?

- Offer a Gift.
- Compose a Gratitude Note.
- Provide a Compliment.
- Craft Something Homemade.
- Invite Her/Them for Coffee.
- Offer a Listening Ear.
- Engage in an Activity They Enjoy.
- Compile a Photo Album.
- Share Some Humor.
- Attend a Movie Together.

Effect of being appreciative in a relationship?

Expressing appreciation motivates your partner to contribute further. It's a form of acknowledgment that doesn't necessarily imply financial constraints but rather signifies respect for your partner's efforts. When you show appreciation, it leaves your partner with smiles, fostering a desire to go above and beyond in their actions and deepen their love for you.

Being appreciative as a child

Frequently, we overlook the contributions of our loved ones, particularly our parents, assuming that their care is a given due to all they've done for us. The most meaningful gift you can offer is showing gratitude for their efforts, conveyed not only through words but also through tangible actions.

Chapter 8

Stress management strategies

Individuals in robust and healthy family relationships often adopt healthier stress coping mechanisms, like confiding in friends and family, steering away from detrimental outlets. This fosters a pattern of collectively addressing challenges, alleviating stress, and discovering effective solutions.

Moreover, stress can influence family relationships by diminishing a person's capacity to engage in family activities or devote adequate attention to their relationships. In certain instances, the physical health repercussions induced by chronic stress may further strain interactions among family members.

What are the ways to manage relationship stress?

- Understand your approach to conflict.
- Pause.
- Engage in a conversation (in person).
- Contemplate the dialogue.
- Consistently assess your own feelings.
- Build connections with others.
- Seek assistance when needed.

Some of these stress relieving activities may work for you, but if not:

Embark on a nature walk, Meditate or engage in yoga, Tend to the garden or undertake a home improvement project, Take a stroll, run, or bike ride to clear your mind. It proves beneficial, believe me.

Things To Do When Your Partner Is Stressed

- Listen without passing judgment and acknowledge their feelings.
- Undertake a few daily actions to ease your partner's life.
- Learn to recognize signs of stress in them.
- Acknowledge that men and women may respond to stress in distinct ways.
- Address the sources of their stress and attempt to alleviate it.

Chapter 9

The Role of Humor in Diffusing Tension

Employing gentle humor often aids in addressing even the most delicate issues.

Humor and laughter have the capacity to open us up, allowing our authentic emotions to surface and enhancing vulnerability. This fosters open communication, intimacy, closeness, and self-regulation, effectively easing tension and conflict. A playful demeanor enables us to tolerate more and reduces defensiveness toward issues that might otherwise cause agitation. This, in turn, promotes learning and a more cooperative spirit.

Humor provides a fresh perspective on issues, fostering creativity in seeking solutions. It alleviates tensions, interrupts power struggles, facilitates reframing, and offers a perspective that deflates anger.

Experiencing stress tightens your body and can induce a feeling of being stuck. A hearty laugh can alleviate physical tension, relaxing muscles for approximately 40 minutes. Additionally, it enhances cardiac health by elevating your heart rate and boosting oxygen levels in your blood.

Engaging in enjoyable activities together fosters positive emotions for couples, leading to increased relationship satisfaction. It helps partners unite to overcome differences and instills hope during challenging times.

Ultimately, having fun presents the opportunity to connect and forge bonds with others. Participating in enjoyable activities not only makes us more pleasant to be around but also creates enduring memories when shared with others, contributing to a lifetime of happiness.

Conclusion

Building a Quarrel-Free Connection

Within the fabric of relationships, where threads of emotion and comprehension intertwine, the quest for a conflict-free connection unfolds as a profound journey.

Navigating the complexities of human connection, this guide transforms into a compass, directing us toward a harmonious destination.

Building a conflict-free connection is not a fixed endpoint but an ongoing dance—a rhythmic partnership where empathy, communication, and shared growth harmonize.

In the concluding notes of this exploration, let us embrace the insight that a conflict-free connection doesn't denote the absence of disagreement but rather signifies the art of resolution.

It encapsulates the alchemy of transforming conflicts into opportunities for understanding and growth.
May the lessons within these pages serve as stepping stones, guiding us through the ebb and flow of relationships, nurturing a space where love, respect, and communication flourish.

As we close this chapter, let the echoes of a quarrel-free connection reverberate in our interactions.

May every disagreement be an invitation to deepen our understanding, and every resolution a testament to the strength of our bonds.

Trying to build a quarrel free home, does not means they will be absent or conflict between parents and child, know this and know peace.

In the ongoing narrative of our connections, may we craft a melody of harmony that resonates through the shared moments of joy, laughter, and enduring love.

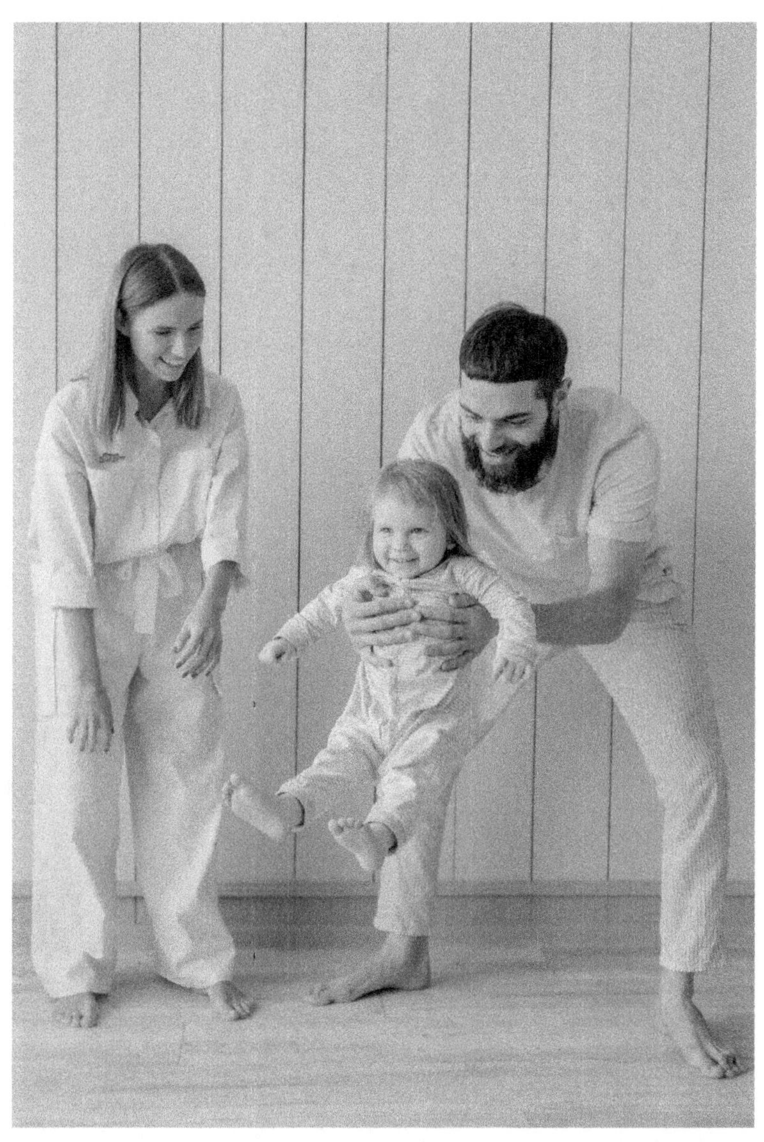